LIVING
a Full and Healthy Life

LIVING

a Full and Healthy Life

Finding Balance
from Within

Darla Lynne Salas

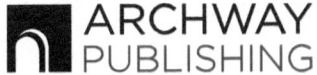
ARCHWAY
PUBLISHING

Scripture quotations are taken from the Holy Bible, New Living Translation, copyright ©1996, 2004, 2007 by Tyndale House Foundation. Used by permission of Tyndale House Publishers, Inc., Carol Stream, Illinois 60188. All rights reserved.

This book is a work of non-fiction. Unless otherwise noted, the author and the publisher make no explicit guarantees as to the accuracy of the information contained in this book and in some cases, names of people and places have been altered to protect their privacy.

Archway Publishing books may be ordered through booksellers or by contacting:

Archway Publishing
1663 Liberty Drive
Bloomington, IN 47403
www.archwaypublishing.com
1 (888) 242-5904

Because of the dynamic nature of the Internet, any web addresses or links contained in this book may have changed since publication and may no longer be valid. The views expressed in this work are solely those of the author and do not necessarily reflect the views of the publisher, and the publisher hereby disclaims any responsibility for them.

Any people depicted in stock imagery provided by Thinkstock are models, and such images are being used for illustrative purposes only. Certain stock imagery © Thinkstock.

ISBN: 978-1-4808-5034-7 (sc)
ISBN: 978-1-4808-5033-0 (hc)
ISBN: 978-1-4808-5035-4 (e)

Library of Congress Control Number: 2017953595

Print information available on the last page.

Archway Publishing rev. date: 10/25/2017

Contents

Acknowledgements

I just want to first thank God for giving me the words to speak and to share what He wants me to say. I would not be where I am today without Him. I also want to thank my husband for standing by my side and supporting me every step of the way. Never a dull moment. For my parents who knew what I had in me and allowing me the space to find it. For all of those that helped me read, re-read, and read it again. You know who you are. Amy, Maria, Anita, Chi Chi, Anna, Judy, Karen, Trish, Laura, Yolanda, and finally The Bridge of Faith family that have always loved and supported me from the beginning.

Darla Salas

Preface

Health as defined by Merriam-Webster, "is the condition of being sound in body, mind, or spirit; flourishing condition." Let's take a look at that a bit further. We think of health as just food and exercise, but it is not. It is so much more than that. It is taking care of your body, and your mind, and your spirit. It is flourishing. It is becoming more that what you are right now. We as women are constantly striving to be more. We are pushing ourselves to fit some standard that the world has set. But that is not what the Lord has required of us. We are to live our lives to serve Him.

I have struggled with my appearance for most of my teen and young adult life. However, there came a point where God showed me what He required from me. Living a healthy and balanced life. Not a life of extremes and diets. But one of joy and peace. One that shows who He is through my lifestyle. I do not claim to be perfect. Only more centered and balanced in Him.

As we progress through this book, remember one thing.

- Psalm 37:5
  Commit everything you do to the Lord. Trust Him to help you to do it and He will.

CHAPTER ONE
Physical Health

PHYSICAL HEALTH. UGH...WHAT A STATEMENT. WE often look in the mirror and think, my physical health needs work. However, when we look at those two words, there are definitions to how we look at physical health. There is not a person on the planet that is 100% happy with their physical appearance. Magazines airbrush, plastic surgeons have waiting lists, and there are make-up stores with a million different options. The world is full of ways to "improve" our physical appearance. Then there is the second word to that, health. Health from taking a million vitamins and other weight loss pills and shakes to working out for hours just to maintain an ideal.

But what does God require of us? We are only given one body here on this earth, so He trusts us to take care of it. We are His masterpiece.

🐦 Ephesians 2:10
For we are God's masterpiece. He has created us anew in Christ Jesus, so we can do the good things he planned for us long ago.

His creation. His temple.

🐦 1 Corinthians 6:19-20
19 Don't you realize that your body is the temple of the Holy Spirit, who lives in you and was given to you by God? You do not belong to yourself, 20 for God bought you with a high price. So you must honor God with your body.

So we are to keep it in good working order. What does that look like? Well, first off, what are we putting in to it? Garbage in...Garbage out. We need to fill our temples with what is going to nourish us and make us grow in a good way.

Food Wise.

We need to be wise in what we take in. The proper way to eat a balanced diet. Now, before we go on, let's define what a diet is. Society says it is a way to eat to lose weight. A restriction of the good stuff. However, Merriam-Webster says it is "food and drink regularly provided or consumed, habitual nourishment." It is what we eat. So to combine the two definitions, society's and Webster's, you either have a good diet or you have a bad diet...either way... you have a diet.

Nutritionists have developed the 'plate'. It is what we should be striving for. It is our balance. Too often when we consume fast food, how do we feel? That burrito at 8 o'clock in the evening? That super-sized combo on the run from one place to another? For the moment our body is satisfied, but then later, we are lethargic and bloated and just plain depressed. Why?? Because we are off balance.

Now let me say, there is nothing wrong with a sweet snack or burger here and there. But there is a difference between that and lifestyle of burgers and shakes.

There is a healthy way to eat. You can use this wherever you go. Picture your plate. Half of it should be Vegetables and Fruits. The other half you will then divide in another half, so a fourth multi grain products, the other fourth protein. Proteins can be soy based like tofu, or meat, poultry, and fish. Then add about a cup of some dairy product. Cheese, milk, or yogurt. Then you want about a fourth of a cup of some healthy fats and oils. An example of a food that is great for this is avocados. Make sure you also consume a lot of water. Even McDonald's offers side salads in place of French fries. It's about being balanced. Eat more fruits and veggies, and there are a lot out there. Try new things. Don't be afraid of all things green. We eat with our eyes first. So...go for colors. Peppers come in all kinds of colors. Red, Yellow, Orange, and they are all sweet. Dip it in some hummus, and there is a great veggie-filled snack. Cauliflower makes a great mashed potato alternative. There are so many options out there. What are some ideas that you know that you can share?

_____

_____

_____

_____

_____

_____

_____

_____

_____

Eating balanced also consists of more than a balanced plate. That's great for once we are home...what about before we get home? Ah...yes...grocery shopping. Getting the goods. There are a few tips to grocery shopping.

1. Never go grocery shopping hungry.
2. Never go grocery shopping tired.
3. Make a list to keep you on task.
4. Don't wander to see what looks good.
5. Stay to the outside.

Now I know this list almost sounds like a sporting event, and in a way, I guess it is. But it is the battle for your health. When you wander in to the grocery store tired and hungry, you will buy what is easy and convenient. You are not going to care about the health factor. You will skip to number 4 and wander to see what looks good. Plan your outing to the market. That leads to planning ahead. Ok... so how do I plan my shopping?

- Start by planning your weekly menu. Get creative. Make it fancy to hang on the wall so all can see what the week holds. Make a calendar to put on the fridge.
- Have a family? Sit down with the kids and come up with dishes that all can enjoy.
- Living alone? Create dishes that you will enjoy cooking for one.
- Have leftovers? Freeze some of it or take it for lunch the next day...or share with someone you know is also alone.
- Make cooking nights with friends. There are a lot of ways you can plan your meals.

What are some options you can think of for meal planning?

_____

_____

_____

_____

_____

_____

_____

_____

_____

So, now you have your meals planned for the week. You have made your list, ate a snack, and are well rested. Let's hit the market. You stay to the outside. Don't wander the inner aisles. The outside is where the fresh fruits and veggies are. All the local and in season produce. The fresh meat and dairy, as well as the whole grain breads. All the wonderful things to make a great and colorful plate. Most cities have farmers markets too, which is a great way to support local growers and get fresh produce. Plus it has the added bonus of getting you out in the fresh air and walking.

Now, what about those nutrition labels??? Those labels are created as ways to help you balance what you eat. You have high blood pressure? Watch that sodium intake. Diabetic? Keep an eye on those carbs and sugars. Wanting to cut down on food consumption in general? Check the servings per container for portion control. The labels are not made to scare you and make you afraid to eat anything. They are there to inform you and to help make you smart about your choices. These labels are like your medicine. You need to watch your doses.

Exercise Vs. Diet

Now that you have your food diet balanced and you have your meal system in place. It is time to bust a move. Yup...move that body. Time to work out!

Again, we are talking about balance. A healthy balance is what we are looking for. Most people do not have 2 hours a day to exercise. Some are doing good to find 10 minutes. But as long as you are making whatever moments you have count...you are moving in the right direction. Doing something for 15 minutes is better than nothing at all. Even if you walk in place in front of the television at night for 30 minutes during the news...or making a game out of *Wheel of Fortune*...you jog when the wheel spins.

Then there is the plank when you get a question wrong on *Jeopardy*...I'd be down there a lot. Not a night person? You prefer morning? Ok...do jumping jacks while you wait for the coffee to brew. Or run in place while the bread is in the toaster. Then there is always the famous "take the last parking spot at work and walk farther"...and taking the stairs to your desk. The whole point is to find healthy movements that fit in to your life. "No matter how slow you go, you are still lapping everybody on the couch." Right now...what small change can you start with?

_____

_____

_____

_____

_____

_____

_____

_____

Now that you're eating better, and have healthy movements throughout the day, make sure you are taking the time to fill up on Jesus.

Challenge yourself to read the Bible in a year. There are several websites that help you break it down. Take a moment, on your lunch break, in the morning with your coffee, or at night as you decompress from your day. There are even those moments in the restroom. The point is… take the time to talk to Him. Stay filled up on His word. We cannot do anything without Him. Sure…we can get a few steps, but I promise you this, you will trip and fall if you are going to try and do it all on your own.

Challenge a woman. Text a sister and see if she read the assigned reading for the day. What did she get out of it? Share what you got out of it. Set up friendly pop quizzes to see who has read that week. Life in the Word is far from boring. Jesus has come to give a full and abundant life. Live it up and celebrate all that we have in Him!!

Eat Healthy-Move Healthy-and Read Healthy.

Balancing your life…one apple, one move, one chapter at a time.

CHAPTER TWO
Heart Health

WHEN WE THINK OF THE HEART...WE THINK OF LOVE and romance. When we think of heart health we think of exercise. However, what about our heart in regards to it belonging to Christ? Is it a place that God wants to live?

Did you know that medically, your heart not only controls both the blood and oxygen flow, but also your well-being mentally? Have you ever been angry? Did you realize that raises your blood pressure? That is not good for the heart. Have you ever held on to that anger? What about being hurt? Have you ever held on to that? That bitterness, that hurt? That physically affects the body. Your joints and muscles tense up and that causes harm to the heart. Holding on to un-forgiveness affects everything about your body. Now, please do not misunderstand the thought that feelings and emotions are wrong, they are not. It is what we do with them that can be our downfall. Jesus was angry in the Temple (**Matthew 21:12-13**). Jesus was also hurt and cried at loss (**John 11:35**). The Bible specifically says

🕊 Ephesians 4:26
   And don't sin by letting anger control you.

Think about it, as you are reading this I know you are thinking about someone that hurt you and did you wrong. You say that you forgive them...but you are not forgetting it. In fact, any chance you get, you tell someone about the wrong that was done to you by someone. I know the words sound easier to say than to do...but LET IT GO!

We have all been there. I know that I have even uttered the words..."Hurt me once shame on you...hurt me twice shame on me." We will talk more in Chapter three on dealing with toxic people and relationships...but what I am wanting to talk to you about is your heart and your heart health.

We need to follow what the Bible says when it tells us to think on the things of Him. Not to focus on the things that have hurt us or have caused a point of contention within our workplace or home. But to think on the things that are worthy of praise.

🕊 Philippians 4:8
And now, dear brothers and sisters, one final thing. Fix your thoughts on what is true, and honorable, and right, and pure, and lovely, and admirable. Think about things that are excellent and worthy of praise.

When we begin to make our focus Him, things will begin to change in our life. When that happens we need to go the next step. We need to learn to hear the heartbeat of God. What does He want for us, our family, our jobs, our church, our neighborhood, our country? God has a plan and a purpose. There is nothing that He does not know.

🕊 Jeremiah 29:11, 13
11-For I know the plans I have for you, says the Lord. They are plans for good and not for evil, to give you a future and a hope.
13-You will find me when you seek me, if you look for me in earnest.

When you look with all your heart to what God truly wants, you will find it...and it is then He can create a new and clean heart. If you are taking the time to eat healthy, have healthy movements, and begin to take care of your physical health, then you need Him to begin to work on the inside as well.

Right now...as you are reading this, take a moment and ask Him. Pray this simple prayer of scripture out loud.

🕊 Psalm 51:7-15

Purify me from my sins, and I will be clean; wash me, and I will be whiter than snow. 8 Oh, give me back my joy again; you have broken me-- now let me rejoice. 9 Don't keep looking at my sins. Remove the stain of my guilt. 10 Create in me a clean heart, O God. Renew a loyal spirit within me. 11 Do not banish me from your presence, and don't take your Holy Spirit from me.12 Restore to me the joy of your salvation, and make me willing to obey you. 13 Then I will teach your ways to rebels, and they will return to you. 14 Forgive me for shedding blood, O God who saves; then I will joyfully sing of your forgiveness 15 Unseal my lips, O Lord, that my mouth may praise you.

If you have junk in your heart and are holding on to bitterness, anger, resentment, grief, pain, you are building a wall between you and Him. Having the emotions is not bad, it is holding on to them and letting them control you that are the bricks. If another person can easily anger you, it is because you are off balance with yourself. It doesn't just affect you. When you are angry at someone, odds are, you take it out on more than just that person. You are mad at your boss, so you bring it home and complain to your spouse, your kids, the dog. Anyone who will listen. But in reality, you are not just "venting" as us women call it...you are spewing toxicity all over the place. You are dumping negative thoughts in to the minds and hearts of those around you.

We as women need to learn, if you want to complain about it...**pray about it!** The next time someone around you starts to spout off about their mother-in-law, neighbor, and co-worker, grab them by the hands and begin praying positivity in to that situation. ***Change the heart.*** After all, you need to **"guard your heart, for it affects everything you do." (Proverbs 4:23)**

Take 10 minutes and write down a few items that you know you struggle with. Be honest with yourself. You are helping NO ONE by holding on to the past. You are the only one preventing yourself from being able to move forward. We already established that God has some great things in store for you...so let the past stay there...in the past.

_____

_____

_____

_____

_____

_____

When you get your heart focused on Jesus and what He wants for you and let go of all the garbage...then love can build and grow. You can begin to walk in peace and freedom. You can then learn all that He has for you.

> 🕊️ James 1:5
> If you need wisdom—if you want to know what God wants you to do—ask him, and he will gladly tell you. He will not resent your asking.

When you are in a relationship...any kind of relationship... it grows and develops because you spend time together. You learn about one another. One of those ways is by asking each other questions. That shows that there is an interest. God would love for you to ask what He wants for you. After all, He created you and put so much in you and in your heart that he is beyond excited to tell you.

Allow your heart to grow. Let go of the past and press on to the future. It is going to be a great one! Fill up on the Word of God. Read His Word and you will hear His heartbeat for you. Listen to worship and praise music. Bring your heart back to what it was created to do...living for Him.

We need to fill our lives with Him. Recently I was struggling with a change in my life. I felt so surrounded by negativity. I began to play praise and worship music and slowly my heart began to change. My situation didn't, my surroundings didn't, but I did. Praise precedes victory. My answer is coming…and my heart is ready.

No matter where you are and what you are doing, technology has evolved that you can always find a way to get the word and worship in to your heart. Find His heart beat and begin drumming. Beating to your own drum will profit you nothing. It will make you loud and noisy and a nuisance to those that are around you.

     I Corinthians 13:1-2
     If I could speak all the languages of earth and of angels, but did not love others, I would only be a noisy gong or a clanging cymbal. 2 If I had the gift of prophecy, and if I understood all of God's secret plans and possessed all knowledge, and if I had such faith that I could move mountains, but didn't love others, I would be nothing.

Beat to His drum with your new heart and worship Him, love Him and grow that healthy heart.

CHAPTER THREE
Relatable Health

RELATIONSHIPS. WHAT A SHIP YARD. YOU HAVE friendships and relationships. You have them with co-workers, family and in-laws. There could be a lot of dinghy's floating out there. So how do you navigate through all of those and find those that are the right ones to anchor down with and which ones you should just open the sails and let float away?

Toxic relationships are easy to spot when someone else is in them. You see them downcast and sad, beaten down and used, always making excuses for their actions...because they love them. Now...take that thought process and think about your own words to others. Do you justify the actions of someone around you? Dr. Steve Maraboli who is a behavioral scientist said this, "If they do it often, it isn't a mistake; it's just their behavior."

- 🐦 Well he doesn't know any better...look at his upbringing.
- 🐦 He's just tired, he works hard.
- 🐦 I made him mad, it was just an accident.
- 🐦 She cares about me, she's just busy and we will get together when she has time.
- 🐦 There was a family emergency and she had to cancel, again.
- 🐦 I said something wrong, it wasn't his fault.
- 🐦 She talks about them that way, but she would never do that to me.

I know personally, I found myself very lonely. I wanted friends and people to like me. So more often than not, I found myself in some very toxic relationships. Not only with men, but with women too. I would change who I was to be liked. I would change my hairstyle, make-up, clothes, and even weight to be liked. I remember a time in the 7th grade when I was at the mall with a girlfriend from church. Before leaving her house, she did my make-up and hair. When we got to the mall she told me to take off my glasses. (I was as blind as a bat...so this could have been bad) Then she informed me that I was her cousin, which made us family so how cool was that. I am now 40, and this event still rings in my head. Why? Because it was toxic. When you have to go to all that work and trouble to have a friend, there is a problem. When you have to fight to be accepted, you already have lost.

You begin to focus so hard on fixing the toxic friendships that you forget about all the people around you that are trying to love you for who you are. "Toxic relationships not only make us unhappy; they corrupt our attitudes and dispositions in ways that undermine healthier relationships and prevent us from realizing how much better things can be."

I recently was in a situation where a huge blessing was trying to come my way. All I needed to do was sit back and relax and let the love come my way. However, I was letting one person and my relationship with her control my surroundings. For the sake of conversation we will call her 'Brenda'. 'Brenda' was someone that I had spent years with and we had grown close. There were even large life events that I had seen her through. But, when I had a large life event happen, it all of a sudden changed things. Up until that point, we were both in the same ship...going the same route. But when all of a sudden, I was upgraded to a cruise ship and not a cargo ship, the water got a bit choppy. I tried so hard to include 'Brenda' in my new journey. To the point where some new passengers on my cruise ship were beginning to wonder what I was thinking. Why was I holding so tightly to something that was clearly not adding a thing to my life? I had a choice to make, I could not hold on to the old cargo and enter the new luxury cruise liner. 'Brenda' and I tried to talk, but she never saw that what she was doing and how she was acting was wrong and hurtful to me. I had to do what was right for me. She told me she was sorry for not being there for me, but it was coated in excuses.

Now don't get me wrong, I read chapter two and I have let the hurt and anger go. But I also learned from this and realized that sometimes, you have to let the old baggage go in order to receive a brand new blessing. Let me tell you, I did. I feel free now to embrace those around me that love me for me and want to be a part of my life.

God wants to bless us with so much more.

There is also the part of our life that is the balancing act. Juggling our time and energy with all that life throws at us. Work and co-workers. Home, family and in-laws. Church, other activities that we are involved in. There are a lot of things that we deal with on a daily basis.

<u>List out a typical day.</u>

Morning—Before work: _____

_____

_____

_____

Morning—At work: _____

_____

_____

_____

Noon Time: _____

_____

_____

_____

Mid-Afternoon—heading home maybe?? _____

_____

_____

_____

Evening: _____

_____

_____

_____

Bed-Time: _____

_____

Tired from thinking about all that? Tired of writing it all out? Tired period??

We as women tend to think of so many things. We have to go here and get this, oh and remind *so-n-so* to get that. I have to email that person, text another and oh yeah... laundry, groceries, meal planning. Nope, nothing going on here.

Balancing is hard work, but we do it all of the time. Balance is defined by Merriam-Webster as "the ability to move or remain in a position without losing control or falling; a state in which different things occur in equal or proper amount of importance." Let that sink in for a moment. Without losing control? Do we lose our cool? Proper amount of importance? Do we have our priorities straight?

We think that if we don't do it, well then, it just won't get done. Simple as that right? Well, what happens if you look at your list and take off just 2 items? Will your day still be ok? What if you look at your list (minus the 2 items) and you now delegate 2 more things? Will your day still go on? The thing with delegating is...you have to let them do it. You have to trust someone else.

When I moved to California and took over the Children's Ministry at my church, I learned a valuable lesson. There were other teachers that could help me and teach. But I wanted them to say what I said and do what I did. However, they were not me. It was the same lesson as I was going to give…they just did it differently. Same result… different path. Just because someone does it differently than you do, does not mean it is wrong. It is just different. Yes, there are wrong, unhealthy ways to cook a chicken, raw for example. However, what if they just decide to bake it and not boil it and make roast chicken soup instead of boiled chicken soup? Is it still soup? Yes. See my point? Delegating means not being in control. We must learn that at the end of the day, we are not in control anyway…God is.

Now back to your list. What else can you delegate and let go of? It's all about making choices and finding balance. Balancing is important. It is about keeping your life on an even flow. Now, I am not saying that this is easy, but it can be done. It is learning what the important things are and prioritizing. It's also an art of taking one day at a time.

What is most important in your life? Fill in your priorities. Number them.

_____

_____

_____

_____

_____

Everyone's list may be slightly different. However, take a moment and compare your list to your typical day list. How does it stack up? The same? Different? What do you see that may need to change? What items might you need to add?

Wrapping up what we know about others, what we know about ourselves, and how to balance it all leads to what honestly and truly matters. What does God require of us?

There are those people that may be in our lives and we say... Lord, I can't take much more of this. Some are blood related, some are work related, and then there are others that we are not sure how they are related. So when we look at who is in our life and what we are dealing with alongside of them or even because of them, ask yourself this: "Lord, do you require this of me?"

Sometimes people are in our lives for a reason. We need to learn something, they need to learn something, or there is a challenge that is needed to overcome on either side. Others are in our lives for a season...a stepping stone to the next phase of what God has for us. They can be there to propel us into the next season that God has planned. Whether that is because they are toxic, or because they pray us in to that next level.

One key thing to help determine their role in your life...is to look at theirs. Are they bearing fruit? Meaning, are they blossoming positivity and peace? Do they encourage you and make you feel better when you are around them? Is it an open two way street with them? Are you leaving them uplifted when they leave your side? Now yes, I do realize that we have bad days. But the scripture has called us to be the salt of the earth (**Matthew 5:13**), and a light, like a city set on a hilltop (**Matthew 5:14**). We are to add flavor to those around us. We are to be a beacon of light in a dark and trying world. We are to show them that through it all, there is hope and peace. A peace that passes all understanding. (**Philippians 4:7**) Again, I state, that this is also a two way street. They are to do the same for us. "As Iron Sharpens Iron." (**Proverbs 27:17**) We are to sharpen one another. Not to make the knife sharp to stab some-one with, but to make them sharper and more prepared for battle in the great big world of unknowns out there.

We need to make sure that the people in our lives are the ones that God wants to keep there. Think about it. Why do you spend time with them? When do you spend time with them? How do you spend time with them?

Why? Is it because you are lonely and have nothing better to do? Is God requiring you to be with them to encourage them and lift them up? Do they lift you up and encourage you in a dark time in your life? Are you bored? Are they bored? Are they lonely and need someone to wallow in self-pity with?

When? Is it only after they have called everyone else and no one is available to hang out and you are the last resort? Are you the first call and it's whenever you both have time because you both know that life happens? Is it when it is only convenient for you and you make them jump through hoops?

How? Do you go out and over spend your budget trying to impress them? Is it going to places that only they like and they never want to go where you want to go and do what you want to do? Is there compromise? Is it all about them? Is it all about you? Is what you both do together uplifting and encouraging to a piece of your health?

These are the things that you look at to decide. It is how you answer the question of what God is requiring of you. Also, people you trust can help. Have you ever had someone tell you that they didn't think that "guy" was good for you? Sure, we all have at some point. So take pause in all your relationships when someone says that. Evaluate it and pray about it. It may be the red flag you needed. But at the end of the day...you live with you. You know deep down inside. Like my example with 'Brenda'...it hurt to walk away from someone I thought was my friend. But I look back now and see blue skies and feel free. God was not requiring me to be a part of that any longer. In fact, He needed me to let go of that and accept the new thing He had in His hand for me.

I leave this chapter with one final thought. Trust the Lord. As we have been talking...you know that He only wants what is best for you.

🦋 Proverbs 3:5-6

Trust in the Lord with all your heart; do not depend on your own understanding.

6 Seek his will in all you do, and he will show you which path to take.

CHAPTER FOUR
Mental Health

MENTAL? I PROMISE, NO CALLING THE MEN WITH THE white coats here. "Am I losing it?" This is something I believe we all ask ourselves occasionally. I promise you are not. But in order to understand our mental state, we need to understand the mind.

There are a many authors out there that you can read all about the mind and the power it possesses. Joyce Meyer, Beth Moore, Rick Warren and Kenneth Copeland. Kenneth Copeland states it beautifully for me, the mind is a battlefield. "The battleground of the mind is where life's most precious victories are won or lost." It is the only place that Satan cannot go. He cannot read your thoughts. He only can tell if the thought that he has placed there is acted upon. Your actions are the only indicator of the battles that rage in your mind.

Let's break this down a bit. If your son, daughter, boss, or anyone else does something that really gets under your skin, how do you react? If you are someone like me, that used to have a real bad temper, probably not well. Now, Satan knew I had a temper and that it would not take much to set me off. My older brother knew this too. You can imagine the poor agony that my mother and father went through with a screaming daughter and a taunting son. You got it. Road trips were a blast!

But you see, I had to learn the Fruit of self-control. My brother had to learn kindness and goodness. My parents were praying for the peace. Because we were all trying to grow in the Fruit of the Spirit, Satan was in an all-out attack mode. If he could get into my head, I could ruin a whole morning with a temper tantrum. Then the whole fruit basket would be upset. He won. That is where the battle begins. In the mind. All Satan has to do is convince you of something. No words need to be spoken. Just a thought that you dwell on.

- 🐦 She looked at me wrong.
- 🐦 Her tone of voice was condescending.
- 🐦 She doesn't do it my way...she's wrong.
- 🐦 Why is he talking to her?
- 🐦 He never called me back.
- 🐦 They're too busy for me...I am just not important anymore.

These are just a few thoughts that I know we struggle with. What are some things that cross your mind that you know are not the truth? Come on...you have those thoughts... and you know full well that they are lies.

_____

_____

_____

_____

_____

_____

_____

_____

_____

🦋 Psalm 139:23
    Search me, O God, and know my heart; test
    me and know my anxious thoughts.

Satan does **NOT CARE ABOUT YOU!** He will play any card he can to get into your head to divide you in pieces. If he can get you out of sorts and focused on something other than what God wants for you, he has won. If he can distract you with other people and their business, he has won.

Worry, Anger, Jealousy, Bitterness, Anxiety, Mistrust, Fear. That list has the same core...Insecurity.

Satan loves using this on us women. If he can get in your head and you think...why did she laugh at what I said? You begin to walk down the road of being overly self-conscious. You are living your life being too sensitive. But that is what Satan needs to divide. If he can get in between a husband and wife and they are arguing on the way to church...then all through service they are not going to be able to receive all that God wants for them. If he can get between any family members during the week, then they are going to be too focused on the problem and not take the time to see what God wants to do in their life.

The thing is, you can choose not to act. If someone looks at you "wrong" in your eyes, stop for a second and re-evaluate. Are they even looking at you or through you because they are focused on another thought? That "tone" they just used...is it possible you read more into it? Instead of getting so offended and thinking that everything is about you take a moment and look at the person. Maybe that person is tired and not feeling well. Maybe they are in a hurry and you stopping them to answer a question was more than what they needed at that

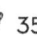

moment. Maybe they were curious and didn't realize that you really didn't want to talk about it. There are a lot of variables. So instead of reacting like Satan is hoping, take a breath and look at the moment. A simple breath can cause a battle to become a moment of conversation and understanding. Come on women...we do have hormones you know. They do fluctuate.

There are several scriptures about the mind and taking our thoughts captive. Take the time to research them. Make them your own.

_____

_____

_____

_____

_____

_____

_____

_____

You need to grab control of yourself and not blame everything that is wrong on someone else. That seems to be
an epidemic lately, and this may be controversial...but
bottom line, people need to take responsibility for their
own actions. Do not blame every bad thing that happens
on others. Sometimes your reactions to someone's look
or tone, that was not even there to begin with, causes a
bigger problem.

Then there is the simple verse in Matthew that says....

🐦 Matthew 18:15
   If another believer sins against you, go pri-
   vately and point out the offense. If the other
   person listens and confesses it, you have won
   that person back.

Go to them...*not to everyone but them*. Bring up the item
that you see that hurt you. But do not go in a way that
is an accusation. Go in a way that shows you are willing
to work it out and have a conversation. Ladies, we are
all adults and should be able to handle someone asking
what we meant by a look or phrase.

Generational Legacy

The definition of legacy is "something that happened in
the past or that comes from someone in the past." Ever
heard the phrase, "The apple doesn't fall far from the

tree"? How about "You are just like your mother."? Well there is more truth to that than you realize. It is your inheritance, your generational legacy.

There was a story once that I heard that a girl was watching her mother make a ham for dinner. She cut the two ends off and put it in the roaster to cook. The daughter inquired why she cut the ends. "My mother always did." The daughter still not satisfied asked why. So she called her mother in to the kitchen and asked her why she did it. The grandmother of the young girl smiled as she was asked and answered, "Well, my mother always did." The granddaughter, still not satisfied asked why. So they all went into the living room where great-grandma was sitting and they asked why she cut the ends off of the ham before cooking it. The old lady smiled and said, "Because the pan I used to own was too small."

So, why do you do the things you do? Was it passed on to you from your parents? Is it a good legacy or a bad legacy? Is it a blessing...or a curse? Is it something that you want to pass on to your children?

I look at the legacy that my grandparents left my parents. Some, I must admit I am very proud to take. The fact that I know Jesus and have a relationship with Him, I am very glad to have that legacy. The fact that my mother is very musically inclined, and has passed that along to me is another attribute I will gladly take. My father's thirst for books and reading...yup take that one too. Look at your life and your parents if you can and list things that you see that you possess that are legacies.

_____

_____

_____

_____

_____

_____

_____

_____

_____

Those are the generational legacies that have been passed down to you. Now, unfortunately there are also the "not so good" things that people inadvertently share as well. Some of the common ones that get passed on are: alcoholism, drugs, and violence. We know that these are things that both men and women see their parents do and have a choice. Are they going to live with the same curse, or are they going to break it and change their future and make their life a blessing? Some that women struggle with that most people don't want to talk about are depression, anxiety, worry, abuse (both physically, mentally and sexually), as well as low self-esteem.

Parents can easily pass these things on to their children. Do me a favor; look at the list of struggles above. Tell me what is the common denominator? You guessed it. Mentality. Now, since we just covered the fact that the mind is a battlefield and we know where some of these thoughts come from, the idea that we can break this cycle should be a bit easier to comprehend.

If you struggle with worry and strife and you get all worked up over not knowing something that honestly doesn't pertain to you, fill that space in your mind with something else. Keep your nose out of other people's business. Do not let the devil get a foothold and cause havoc in your mind. If you get depressed easily and are not sure why, again… fill your mind with the Word and remove the thoughts that the devil is trying to place there. It is the first step to breaking the generational curse.

I love my mother and her mother, but I know that the era that my grandmother was raised in, put things on women that didn't need to be there. My mother broke some of those as to not put them on me. As time progresses, I see things in me that I don't want to pass on. Now, I do not have children to "pass" things on to, but I do have young women that are around me. It is my responsibility as a woman of God to show them who He is in me. Remember, we are salt and light. So keep that in mind when you think that this does not apply to you…because it does.

So, when you look at your habits and your mind, realize you are the holder of your mental health. You can control what you think and what you do. Take a breath before reacting. Take responsibility for your own actions. Deal with conflict the Biblical way and not by spreading gossip. Keep your nose out of other people's business. You do not have to know everything about everyone. It is not always about you. Break the generational things in your family and be free from oppression. "When we will our thoughts with right things, the wrong ones have no room to enter." Joyce Meyer is right, an empty space is vulnerable to the enemy settling in.

If you want to begin to pray away those things in the past but are unsure of how to begin…start with how Jesus taught us to pray. Pray that His will and desires for you will be done. That He will help you forgive those that may have hurt you. Pray that He will keep you from the temptations that the enemy tries to set in your mind. It is such a simple prayer to pray, but it holds so much power. You are asking for His very kingdom to come to you here on earth and to show you a new and healthier way to live in Him. Pray for the next phase of your health to flourish.

Our Father
Who art in Heaven, hallowed be
Thy name. Thy Kingdom come,
Thy will be done on earth,
as it is in Heaven. Give us this day
our daily bread. And forgive us
our debts, as we forgive our debtors.
And lead us not into temptation,
but deliver us from evil.
For Thine is the Kingdom,
and the power and
the Glory forever.
Amen.

Matthew 6: 9-13
21st Century KJV

CHAPTER FIVE
Emotional Health

YOU CANNOT HONESTLY DEAL WITH YOUR MENTAL health without it flowing in to your emotional health. Every human has what they call an emotional intelligence. It is what causes you to feel and express what you are feeling. Being aware of your emotions and how you handle them is your EI, (Emotional Intelligence). That stems to also taking responsibility for your emotions. Your Emotional Intelligence is linked to being emotionally self-aware. Emotional self-awareness is knowing what one is feeling at any given time and understanding the impact those moods have on others. It has four branches. Understanding Emotions, Using Emotions, Managing Emotions, and Perceiving Emotions.

It is ok to be angry. But the Bible says to be angry and sin not.

🐦 Ephesians 4:26-27
And "don't sin by letting anger control you." Don't let the sun go down while you are still angry, 27 for anger gives a foothold to the devil.

The scripture never says that anger is wrong. It says do not sin by letting your anger control you. It is a normal human emotion to get hurt, to get mad, and to be frustrated. You can go through the emotions...over the river and even through the woods. But it is what you do when you get to grandmother's house.

Now, I know we are all perfect right? Therefore, I know that we have never said anything in anger. So dealing with this "emotions thing" is no problem right? Wrong. We all have emotions that we struggle with. I have listed mine. What are some things that you struggle with?

_____

_____

_____

_____

_____

_____

_____

_____

_____

_____

"Anyone can be angry-that is easy. But to be angry with the right person, to the right degree, at the right time, for the right purpose, and at the right way-that is not easy."

—Aristotle.

It is so easy for us as women to bottle up our emotions and act like it is all ok. We feel the need to impress and have it all together. Then there are other women that open those bottles and pour everyone around them a big, tall glass and share it. Again, we need to find the balance from within. It is about praying through our emotions. There are times when it is completely understandable to be hurt and angry. There are times it is an acceptable and even a bit on the healthy side to be afraid. In a parking garage at night is one of them. It is what keeps you aware of your surroundings. Stress is an emotion that does not aid in your body's normal balance. In fact, if you speak to most physician's they will tell you about Cortisol levels. Cortisol is a hormone that when increased due to stress, has negative reaction to your body.

According to Dr. Axe, here are some.

- Weight Gain-Especially around the abdomen/stomach
- Puffy, Flushed face
- Mood Swings
- Increased Anxiety
- Fatigue/Poor Sleep
- Increased Urination
- Irregular Periods & Fertility Problems
- Higher Susceptibility to Infections
- High Blood Pressure
- Acne/Changes in the skin
- Higher Risk for Bone fractures
- Muscle Aches & Pains
- Changes in Libido
- Excessive thirst

Women, we have to get a grip on our emotions. We have to live a real and balanced life. Part of the emotional imbalance is we are trying to do too much. We talked about this already. Do what you can to keep your mind intact. When your mind becomes more stable, your emotions should start to follow. When your emotions start to balance out, you will notice that you will start to feel better.

You can ask almost any doctor, your emotions will affect your physical health. You can exercise in the gym two hours a day and eat healthy. However, if you are holding on to anger and hurt, if you are stressed about bills and are afraid for your marriage or job, your body could begin to feel the effects of the stress in certain areas.

- Anger-Weakens the liver
- Grief-Weakens the lung
- Worry-Weakens the stomach
- Stress-Weakens the heart and brain
- Fear-Weakens the kidney

Ladies, take a moment...think. What are you stressed about? What weighs heavy on your mind? Write them down.

_____

_____

_____

_____

_____

_____

_____

_____

Now let us take a moment and see what the Bible says about worry and stress.

🐦 Philippians 4: 6-7

6 Don't worry about anything; instead, pray about everything. Tell God what you need, and thank him for all he has done. 7 Then you will experience God's peace, which exceeds anything we can understand. His peace will guard your hearts and minds as you live in Christ Jesus.

These verses of scripture talk about your heart from chapter two, your mind from chapter four and it tells you how to live in peace. Trust in God. Tell Him what you need. He knows it, but like any good, growing relationship, you need to tell Him. He needs to hear from you. If you are worried about work, your marriage, your children, your income, tell Him. There is nothing that He would not do for you. You are His child and He sent His only Son to this earth to pay the biggest price so that you could spend eternity with Him.

Living worry free and stress free is not always easy, but like I mentioned before, being real plays a part in that. When we are not always trying to live up to the "Jones'" and we are not trying to impress others...it takes some of the pressure off.   If you have managed to do what we talked about in chapter three and remove some of those toxic relationships, and you are not having to pretend anymore, that will help. If you have gone through your generational legacy and removed the curses of depression, anger and strife and are living a blessed filled life that too will help. Often times, we as women are real good to add additional stress and pressure to our life because of expectations we place on ourselves.

Let me clarify, there is nothing wrong with setting goals and dreams for yourself, but just be wary that you are not setting someone else's expectations on yourself. Be who God called you to be. You have to be real with yourself, before you can be real with anyone else. Margery Williams gives a great example of being real in her book *The Velveteen Rabbit*. It is what God wants of us.

> "Real isn't how you are made,' said the Skin Horse. 'It's a thing that happens to you. When a child loves you for a long, long time, not just to play with, but REALLY loves you, then you become Real.'
>
> 'Does it hurt?' asked the Rabbit.
>
> 'Sometimes,' said the Skin Horse, for he was always truthful. 'When you are Real you don't mind being hurt.'
>
> 'Does it happen all at once, like being wound up,' he asked, 'or bit by bit?'

'It doesn't happen all at once,' said the Skin Horse. 'You become. It takes a long time. That's why it doesn't happen often to people who break easily, or have sharp edges, or who have to be carefully kept. Generally, by the time you are Real, most of your hair has been loved off, and your eyes drop out and you get loose in the joints and very shabby. But these things don't matter at all, because once you are Real you can't be ugly, except to people who don't understand."

—Margery Williams Bianco,
The Velveteen Rabbit

Being real is a thing that happens to you. And yes, sometimes it hurts. No, it doesn't happen all at once. It is a process. It is when we grow and change and become more like Christ. You have to be someone that doesn't break easily and you can't have sharp edges that go around poking everyone. But to those that love you and truly accept you, you can be real.

Being real means you have your mind in the right place. Your heart is focused on what God wants for you. You have the people in your life that are supposed to be there and will continue to lift you up on your journey. You have cast off the curses and evil thoughts that have been trying to ensnare you. You are exercising and eating better. You are now living a balanced and full life. You are comfortable in your skin, so you can begin to be real with others.

You can be the emotional support to someone that needs that extra hug. You are now able to see who to pour more salt on to add flavor to their life and who to shine more light on to get them out of a dark time.

CHAPTER SIX

Spiritual Health

OUR SPIRITUAL HEALTH IS PARAMOUNT TO OUR balance. If we are not spending time with God on a daily basis, we become agitated quickly, overwhelmed easily, and lost mentally and emotionally. We spent the last two chapters discussing our mental and emotional health and how to find the balance within them, but as Christian women, that is directly linked to our spiritual health as well. When you are completely in tune with what God is telling you and with what His will is for your life, you are in harmony and balance with yourself. Let us be honest with ourselves. We are not always in that situation are we? We miss a devotion. We say a rushed prayer in the car, or at a stop light on our way to an appointment. There is nothing wrong with those, but that cannot be all that we do outside of a Sunday morning service.

I know that I used to be a night owl. Now I cannot stay up past 9:30 or 10:00pm. Our lives change. We must learn to change and adapt as well. Evening devotional time does not work for me anymore. Getting up in the morning and sharing a house and room, I cannot do my devotions first thing in the morning either. My mental 'peak' if you will, is mid-morning. So that is when I take the time to do my conversing. We had discussed that our relationship with God is like other relationships. You need to invest in it, especially if it is going to grow and succeed.

What is your best time of day? When do you have the most private and quiet time? When is the time that you are alert and not falling asleep in the middle of a conversation?

_____

_____

_____

_____

_____

_____

_____

_____

Stepping in Season

The Bible tells us that we should be ready in season, out of season, in every season. Let me explain. In season is when we are ready for whatever the Lord is going to bring our way. The good, prosperity, joy, and peace. We are ready. The blessings can flow on down. But what about when the blessings don't flow on down. What if something else flows our way? What if nothing comes our way? The river just dries up? No water, no flowers, just a whole lot of manure. Are you ready for that too? Are you so in tune with God that you will be ready to stand when the wind is blowing you in the face and rain is pouring down? Do you have the know-how to stand up to the waves that are rocking your boat and say..."Peace be still." That is being ready out of season. It is having the kind of relationship where even though you do not see His hand moving and you are unsure of the next step, you know that there is another step coming. You know that there will be solid ground, and that is found in our rock, Jesus Christ.

I heard a friend once say, "It is not for me to understand what God is doing, it is for me to trust that He is doing something." What a way to live. That is being ready in season and out of season. That is every season. That is living a fruit filled, spirit led life. It is trusting that in every season we know that He is still God. By being ready in what ever season He places us, we show who He is in and through us. What a better testimony than our lives. When people who do not know who Jesus is, see us go through tough times and not get all out of whack, they wonder. Where does that peace come from? How is she still so sane? What is it about her that she can still do all that she is doing and not drown?

We are starting a new life. We have begun to get our physical health back, we are mentally and emotionally stronger, and we have changed and cleaned our hearts and our lives from toxic relationships. We should be in the best place in our life to embrace the new season we are beginning to walk in to.

I have waited for over 20 years to begin to get the strength up to walk in my new season. I lived in fear for so long. Fear of failure, rejection, and judgment. But I have a new me. I am getting my heart, mind, emotions and life in alignment with what God is doing! You too have a decision to make. Are you ready to take the 'right' exit and go down a road to the new you? The you that is going to grow in Him? Make a change. Right now write down 3-5 things that you are going to do to become more about Him and less about you. Think past your own fears and failures. Think about His love and His kingdom and what He can do through you.

_____

_____

_____

_____

_____

_____

_____

_____

I want to share about two women that you may or may not know about. The first is a woman named Ruth. Her husband died, and she was living alone with her mother-in-law. This woman could have gone home with her parents and started over again. But she didn't. She was ready for a new season. When her mother-in-law said she was leaving and going back to her home town, Ruth said that she was going too. She lost her husband, the man that she loved more than anything. But yet, she says to her mother-in-law, that she will go where she goes, that her people will become her people and that the God that has shown them mercy, will be the same God that she will follow. She embraced a new season.

The second woman that I want to introduce you to is Esther. We meet Esther as a little Jewish girl named Hadassah. She was taken as a young girl in to the palace, with many other young girls, to be a possible replacement to the queen. What kind of King are you going to be married to? However, Esther kept herself humble. She embraced her new season. God needed her to be ready. For it was because of her that she saved all the Jews in the Persian Empire. Imagine if she had been out of season and chose to let her emotions control her circumstance.

🖋 Esther 4:4
Perhaps this is the moment for which you have been created.

Read the book of Esther and Ruth. Think about what they went through. Would you have done the same?

Thoughts?

_____

_____

_____

_____

_____

_____

_____

_____

_____

It is through these women that we can learn to grow in Christ. Through His word. Through our faith and trust in Him. Through the fellowship of other women. We as women can so easily tear other women down. From how they are dressed, to their weight, where they live or don't live. What kind of education do they have? Imagine though…just for a moment…that we all love and support one another, and if we don't agree, we pray about it. That is a sweet season to live in.

So ladies…as we continue to grow. Be ready!
In season.
Out of season.
And for a new season.

CHAPTER SEVEN
Happy Health

WHEN SOMEONE ASKS YOU WHAT MAKES YOU HAPPY, what is the first thing that comes to mind? When you are asked where do you like to go, where is your happy place? What is your dream vacation? Doing everything that you love...with the perfect person. What does that look like?

_____

_____

_____

_____

_____

Alright, you have defined your perfect vacation, with the perfect person, doing your perfect things. Now wake up! You are living here in the real world where work and life and responsibilities are waiting for you from the moment you wake up to the moment you lay your head back down.

But wait a minute. Aren't we learning to live a full and healthy life? Are we not to live a balanced life? What about what I like to do verses what I have to do? Well, that is what could be defined as Happy Health. Merriam-Webster defines happy as "notably fitting, effective, or well adapted, enjoying or characterized by well-being and contentment, expressing, reflecting, or marked by an atmosphere of good fellowship."

Notably fitting? Effective? Well adapted? I would not have thought those to be words to describe happy. However, if we are to find happiness and balance, then those have to be our definitions. We need to find things in our lives that make us effective. When we work, our paycheck makes us effective. We work because we need the income right? When we are balanced in our home life and with work, we become a well-adapted woman. Meaning that we are tolerable to live with.

I don't know about you, but I want more for my life than just being tolerable. I want to be notably fitting. I want to be someone that others take notice of. Now, I am not saying that we are all to become divas and self-centered.

I am saying that we need to be happy and content in our minds, emotions, in our physical health, spiritually, and in our relationships with others. It is there where we can be free to do what makes us happy.

For some that is music. Singing, playing an instrument, dancing. Others may like to be more low key and love to read a good book in a quiet room with a cup of tea. Then there are those who love to go out. Those that work out. Some are more creative. The point is we all have talents that God has given us, and we need to take a time-out and rejuvenate ourselves in our happy place.

- Movies
- Sewing/Quilting
- Swimming
- Crafting
- Music/Instrument
- Photography/Photos
- Painting/Art
- Writing/Reading
- Gardening/Flowers
- Cooking/Baking

What is your passion? What makes you happy? What is your REAL happy place?

_____

_____

_____

_____

_____

_____

_____

_____

George Bernard Shaw was quoted and makes a great point. "Life isn't about finding yourself. Life is about cre-ating yourself." People often say "I need to find myself." You already have. You truly know yourself. You know what makes you mad, sad, and hurt. You know how to deal with your mind and your heart. You know that you get cranky when you are tired. You get moody when you need a meal. What is your next step? It is taking the time to get to know your happy self.

As a woman, the older I got the more I felt like I was not going to measure up to society's version of what I should be. You know that version:

- Twenties you marry and have a family. After going to college of course.
- Thirties you spend supporting your kids and husband and their activities.
- Forties/Fifties you find a job to keep you occupied until grandbabies.
- Sixties/Seventies you retire and enjoy the grandchildren and travel.

Forget that maybe you don't fit that mold. I didn't, and I know I am not the only one. So what do you do when the world around you is trying to squeeze you into its mold?

- Romans 12:12
  Don't copy the behavior and customs of
  this world, but let God transform you into a
  new person by changing the way you think.
  Then you will learn to know God's will for you,
  which is good and pleasing and perfect.

It is time to create yourself. Let what you love to do in your heart guide you. God put things in you, creative things. Not just one thing, but several. There are people who say,

I am not talented. NOT TRUE! It just takes time to discover your creative side. What are you creative with and what do you enjoy?

_____

_____

_____

_____

_____

_____

_____

_____

I do want to touch on one thing. That is the difference between gifts and talents. Here is a list that I found that gives a great explanation.

Talents Vs. Gifts

<u>Natural Talents:</u>
- 🕊 From God through parents.
- 🕊 From birth.
- 🕊 To benefit mankind on a natural level.
- 🕊 Must be recognized, developed, and exercised.
- 🕊 Ought to be dedicated by believers.

<u>Spiritual Gifts:</u>
- 🕊 From God independent from parents.
- 🕊 From rebirth.
- 🕊 To benefit mankind on the spiritual level.
- 🕊 Must be recognized, developed, and exercised.
- 🕊 Ought to be used for God, by God, for His Glory.

There are talents, everyone has those. There are also gifts, and we all have those too. It is just a matter of finding what those are and walking in them.

Listing of Spiritual Gifts:

<u>Romans 12</u>		<u>I Peter 4</u>	
Encouragement	Giving	Serving	Teaching
Leadership	Mercy		
Prophecy	Service		
Teaching			

I Corinthians 12

Administration	Apostle
Discernment	Faith
Healing	Helps
Interpretation	Knowledge
Tongues	Miracles
Prophecy	Teaching
Wisdom	

Ephesians 4

Apostle	Evangelism
Pastor	Prophecy
Teaching	

If you are not sure exactly what your gifting is, pray about it. God will begin to reveal things in you. Do not be afraid to try new things. Disney's Pixar creators believe that if their staff is not failing, then they are not trying new things. Therefore, we should not fear failure, it is just an indicator of what works and does not work. It is embracing the creative process within you and developing your happy place. "Your talent is God's gift to you, what you do with it is your gift back to God."

🖋 1 Peter 4:10
God has given each of you a gift from His great variety of spiritual gifts. Use them well to serve one another.

As the previous page shows there is a difference between what you are talented with and what you are gifted in. The point of this chapter that I want to emphasize, is find something that is yours. What makes you happy? What brings you joy? Find those things and do them. It is what helps bring balance to your life. It fills your life so that you might live a full and balanced life in Jesus.

CHAPTER EIGHT
Financial Health

FINANCES. SOUNDS ABOUT AS EXCITING AS A ROOT canal right? Well, it can be. That is the joy of being healthy and balanced in all areas of your life. When you have things in order, a root canal can be avoided. It is all on how you want to define it. For example, we looked at the words diet and health and happy. Not the definitions we originally thought about right? Why? Because society has changed and skewed the way we look at things. So, to define the previous chapters, it is saying that we are living our life on a budget. We are budgeting our physical health, our emotions, our heart, our relationships, our mental state, and our happiness. Budgeting by definition is "a plan for the coordination of resources and expenditures." That is what we are learning to do in our lives. We are making a plan for our future and for the new seasons in our lives. We are taking the resources that we are receiving and coordinating them. Making the necessary changes and allowances for the expenditures.

So yes, ladies, we can live a healthy life on a budget!! We can adjust our income to do a few things. First, and foremost, honor God. Second, make sure our priorities are met. Third, save a little for a rainy day, and fourth, LIVE! I know you are thinking that it is easier said than done. No, it's not. It just takes knowledge and discipline. But, hey, we are putting our lives in order so that our lives can be full. So, let's fill it up!

What are some things you would like to do with your life? Travel? Buy a house? Get a new car? Start a business? Bless your kids with a good education? Bless your grand-kids? We all have goals and dreams. List a few of the things that you would love to do.

_____

_____

_____

_____

_____

_____

_____

_____

_____

So the first step in dealing with a budget and finances is to look at them. Where is all of my money going? How am I spending my paycheck? Before online banking, most of us would use the check registers and see what we wrote our checks for. Now, we use a debit card...see our balance on our phone...and as long as there is money, we buy.

So, if you are wanting to create a budget to save for say a trip, you have to first know where your money is going to know where to trim the fat. So, sit down at your computer or where ever you can access your funds and make a list. I will help you start.

- 🕊 Tithe: _____
- 🕊 Rent/Mortgage: _____
- 🕊 Insurance: _____
- 🕊 Car: _____
- 🕊 Gas: _____
- 🕊 Cell Phone: _____

You can fill in the rest with what you pay. *Be honest* and do the math.

_____

_____

_____

_____

_____

_____

_____

_____

_____

Are you feeling the squeeze? I was surprised how much I spent on some things and others I was shocked at how little. Getting married made a big difference. But it was a good difference for both my husband and I. When you are single, you only have to account where your money goes for yourself. But when you are married, there is an accountability that *should* come in to play.

Now...this is not a bad thing. It is a way to make you think about what you are spending the income on. I will use my marriage as an example. My husband loves his guitars and truck. I love books, shoes and purses. (You can already see what is coming right?) I don't want to begrudge him the joy of buying things for his truck and he doesn't want to make me feel like I can't have a nice pair of cute shoes. So, we budget. We plan. We wait for sales. We go to truck shows where they bundle items for great deals and packages. It's making smart decisions with what you have to enjoy life. Just because you are on living "on a budget", doesn't mean you are depriving yourself from going anywhere or doing anything. It's being aware and making smart decisions. For example, I wanted to do an activity with my mother and sister while they were visiting over a Christmas break. So I found a coupon that charged us $22.00/ person instead of the full price of $49.00. Yes, it takes a little more effort to look for the sales and deals. But at the end of the month when you have $27.00 extra you feel accomplished. There is the rainy day fund contribution.

The second part to having accountability is also having that person in it with you. My husband and I want to travel. We have an extensive list of places we want to go. But to us, it is not a far off someday. We are making plans and budgeting together. We have a common goal, therefore, we have a common accountability. Do I need those new shoes right now...or can I wait and put this money toward our trip? And he can ask me that without me being offended?

So now we have learned what a budget is, where our money is going and how to better save it right? Smart decisions and being aware of what we are doing. So now I want to go over the most important aspect of our financial health.

Tithing. Now some say, well I put money in the plate, isn't that enough? Well, to be blatantly honest, no it is not. Tithing is the conscious decision that you are going to take the first tenth of your income and give it back to God.

🐦 Deuteronomy 14:23
Bring this tithe to the designated place of worship...doing this will teach you always to fear the Lord your God.

That is all He is asking for. Think about it. If you have a dollar, all He is asking for is 10 cents.

🐦 Numbers 18:26 & 28
26 Give a tenth of the tithes you receive—to the Lord as a sacred offering.
28 ...This is the Lord's sacred portion...

It is only right to give to Jesus what truly He has given to us. Think about the job that you have, the car you drive, the house you live in. That is all of God's doing. He is the one that provides for us. He is Jehovah Jireh. Translated that means He is 'Our Provider'. He is the one that provides for our every need.

Now, when talking about tithing, it is more than just saying, "Well here then Lord, here is your 10%." It is about being joyful about our giving. We need to be open and grateful when we give. After all, it is all His and He is only asking for a tenth.

- 2 Corinthians 9:6-7
  6 Remember this—a farmer who plants only a few seeds will get a small crop. But the one who plants generously will get a generous crop. 7 You must each decide in your heart how much to give. And don't give reluctantly or in response to pressure. "For God loves a person who gives cheerfully."

It needs to be more than that for us. It needs to become a part of who we are. Not just our tax write off, or because everyone is looking at who is putting money in an envelope. We are longing to live a full and blessed life and it is what spiritually we know we are to do. It is all about Him. It is about honoring Him. Think about the law of reaping and sowing. If you are holding on to what is God's, how can He bless you with more? You need to let go of what is asked, and you will see Him open the floodgates of heaven and pour out wonderful and great blessings upon you. Honor the Lord with your physical body, your mind, your heart, your emotions, and spiritually give Him all of who you are. To be full, give him your finances too and watch what He will do.

So as we wrap up the conversation about financial health, located on the next page is a weekly budget sheet that you can use if you like to get a better grip on your finances. I am also leaving you with what I have been striving for that I learned in a Marriage and Family Class on Finances. It is from Dave Ramsey. It is seven simple steps to being financially free. Some may or may not apply to you. However, the ideas and principles are there to start a solid foundation.

<u>DAVE RAMSEY'S SEVEN BABY STEPS</u>

1. $1,000 Emergency Fund
2. Pay off all debt-Debt Snowball
3. Three to six months of expenses in savings
4. Invest 15% of household income into Roth IRS and pre-tax retirement
5. College funding for children
6. Pay off home early
7. Build wealth and give

List your steps:

_____

_____

_____

_____

_____

_____

CHAPTER NINE
Educational Health

WE ARE NEVER TOO OLD TO STOP LEARNING. AS children grow up we make sure to stress the importance of a good education to them. High School, Trade Schools, College, Master's programs, and even Ph.D.'s. So what makes us think that the process of learning and being educated should end and not apply to us as "adults". We push education on "kids" younger than us as if we have hit this magic age of no longer needing to learn. Who says that? Who taught that? Is it the "I'm too old to be in college" thought? College costs money? Well what if I told you that libraries are free and full of information and as long as you are on this earth you are still filling your mind. The question should be, with what?

I know personally that when I went to England through a Study Abroad Program, it was the most terrifying thing yet most exciting thing that I have ever done. I learned. That is the key. I learned about myself, the world around me, about other cultures and lifestyles, and about other generations. I was the oldest in our group of 30, and that included the professor that came with our school.

When I say that I learned about myself, I learned to be alone with myself. That is not always easy for everybody to do. I learned about my insecurities and my fears. It made me stronger. I learned about the world around me, in England. Yes, I have lived in 4 different states and traveled the United States a lot in my first 20 years. I had seen that things are not always the same. Culture and demographics change a lot from coast to coast. However, that would never prepare me for outside our continent. How the world views Americans for instance is eye opening. Sometimes it was downright embarrassing. Nonetheless, I was educated about some things in the world around me. I tasted some great food, tried on some great fashions and learned a different lifestyle. Lastly, I learned about the younger generation and how they view life, politics and religion. How they travel and live life with such abandon.

How do we live? We live such responsible and respectable lives. Taking care of our families, working our jobs and paying our bills. Now, please do not misinterpret that phrase as an insult. It is not. It is our life. We are living it full and balanced and we are finding joy in every aspect. That is what I want to make sure that we all understand. To keep growing and learning. Knowledge is power. It gives us the tools we need to get to a better place. With education we cannot allow anyone to dictate how we live and what we are to do. We know better and are more informed about situations that surround us. With education you can take off the dunce cap and stop pleading ignorance.

We are women that are strong and self-assured. We have our physical bodies in shape. We are eating healthy and exercising. We have our thoughts and emotions in line with our spirit and all that is in tune with God. We have our heart right and are living a happy and fun-filled life. We are not to be belittled and talked down to. We are not to be stuck in a corner and told to hush. In the words of Patrick Swayze, "Nobody puts Baby in the corner."

My point is ladies, we are to keep our minds sharp and exploring educational avenues is paramount to that. I understand that not everyone can enroll in college classes. However, you can go to a Bible Study. You can become a part of a church group that is teaching on a particular subject that interests you. The internet makes it easy too. There are plenty of avenues out there to go down chasing the multifaceted ways to educate yourself.

Think about it. What are some topics that you are interested in learning about? It does not have to be just Bible based. I am asking in any area. Write them down.

_____

_____

_____

_____

_____

_____

_____

_____

_____

I challenge you right now to list a few books that you can read to educate yourself in the topics you just listed. Take the time to do some research and see what is out there. Ask some friends that may know. Right now...make that list and take that step.

_____

_____

_____

_____

_____

_____

_____

_____

_____

You will begin to see and feel a new challenge to your life. The joy of learning something new. A newer and stronger you will begin to emerge. Now, I want to specify one thing. This is not the same as learning a new craft, or something creative...although you can read and learn those things too. However, this is more of a challenge to grow the big grey thing inside your head. Grow your Mind!!

🕊 Proverbs 15:2
   The wise person makes learning a joy; fools spout only foolishness.

I do want to discuss educating ourselves in the Word. Reading the Bible through in a year is one way to learn. It encourages you to stay focused on what God is telling you. It is vital to stay planted near His streams. It is by His water that we can be refreshed and nourished.

🕊 Psalm 1:3
   They are like trees planted along the river-bank, bearing fruit each season. Their leaves never wither, and they prosper in all they do.

Think for a moment, what feeds a tree? Water. So if Psalms tells us to be planted like a tree near the riverbank, we should be growing. Learning His word and develop a knowledge of His plan and His purposes for our life.

Through these past chapters, we have discussed what a few of those are. Remember?

_____

_____

_____

_____

_____

_____

_____

_____

We are to be growing in Him. That way we can maintain our fruit, no matter what the season is. That is the power of educating ourselves with His word.

Knowledge is power. We know that.

His power in us is what makes us strong. His knowledge is what guides us. It is His love that governs us. His grace and mercy keeps us. All of who He is in us is what makes us the strong and beautiful women that we are today. Hold on to Him and His word. Grow in it...you beautiful woman of God.

CHAPTER TEN
Health Abroad

THERE IS NOTHING MORE EXCITING THAN PLANNING A vacation. Especially when you have the funds. Not to mention you get free luggage check in and you get to fly first class. Plus, you are not going alone. Best vacation ever right? However, I have not told you where you are going yet. Are you still excited? What about what you are going to do when you get to this unknown destination...that you can't pack for because again...destination unknown.

Now what? Well, that is where faith comes in. You take what you know and step out. You know that it is all paid for right? You know that you are flying first class, and free check in on luggage. You know you will not be alone. That is your life. Yes sir-ee! You have a full and balanced life. Now take it somewhere, and take someone with you.

Over the last nine chapters we have discussed all the ways to balance our lives to live them to the fullest and healthiest. We have our physical health in check. We are exercising and eating healthier. We are focused on God's Word and have our hearts beating to His drum. The people that are in our lives are welcome there. Our minds and emotions are in line with our hearts and spirit. We are developing new areas of our lives creatively and are using the gifts and talents that He gave us. Money? No problem, we have that in check and have even begun to learn new things. All that we have left to do now, is to share our fruit with others.

That's right. Take a journey outside of your world and share what you have learned with others. Think about who is in your life that can use a little balance. Maybe they need a toxic person intervention. Maybe their talent is buried and they need help finding it. You have your passport. Use it.

Who can you help and how?

_____

_____

_____

_____

_____

_____

_____

_____

_____

_____

I want to share with you a quote by Charles Spurgeon. Think about what you have that you can share with the world. Let me remind you that we are called to be salt to the world and light, a city set on a hill.

> Show the world that your God is worth ten thousand worlds to you. Show rich men how rich you are in your poverty when the Lord God is your helper. Show the strong man how strong you are in your weakness when underneath you are the everlasting arms.
> —Charles Spurgeon

God has blessed us more than what we truly deserve. It is in and through Him that we are even still here. Our sins should have taken us out a long time ago. However, God has a plan for us. We now have a better understanding of what that is. "As you get older, you will start to understand more and more that in life, it's not about what you look like or what you own, it's all about the person you've become." Wouldn't it be great for everyone to live in that freedom?

Remember Who You Are

- A daughter of the King   Galations 3:26
- God-Fearing Woman   Proverbs 31:30
- Steadfast in the love of Christ   Romans 8:31-38
- Redeemed   Ephesians 1:7
- Bought with a price   Isaiah 43:3
- Worth more than precious rubies   Proverbs 31:10
- More than make-up and clothes   I Peter 3:3-4
- Free   John 8:36
- Worth it   Romans 5:6-8
- Victorious   Philippians 4:13
- Joyful   John 15:11
- Transformed   Romans 12:2
- Dignified   Proverbs 22:11
- Favoured   Proverbs 8:35

References

"Aristotle Quotes." *BrainyQuote*. Xplore, n.d. Web. 12 Jan. 2017. <https://www.brainyquote.com/quotes/authors/a/aristotle.html>.

Axe, Josh. "Dr. Josh Axe." *Facebook - Log In or Sign Up*. Dr. Axe., n.d. Web. 12 Jan. 2017.

Bianco, Margery Williams, and Florence Graham. *The Velveteen Rabbit, Or, How Toys Become Real*. New York: Platt & Munk, 1987. Print.

"BibleGateway." *BibleGateway.com: A Searchable Online Bible in over 150 Versions and 50 Languages*. New Living Translation, n.d. Web. 12 Jan. 2017.

Copeland, Kenneth. "One-Year Bible." *Kenneth Copeland Ministries*. Eagle Mountain, n.d. Web. 12 Jan. 2017. <http://www.kcm.org/read/one-year-bible>.

"Dictionary." *Merriam-Webster*. Merriam-Webster, n.d. Web. 12 Jan. 2017.

Goleman, Daniel. "Emotional Intelligence." *Daniel Goleman*. Bantam Books, n.d. Web. 12 Jan.

2017. <http://www.danielgoleman.info/topics/emotional-intelligence/>.

LeLaCheur, Dan. *Generational Legacy*. Eugene, Or.: Family Survival, 1994. Print.

Maraboli, Steve. "Steve Maraboli Quotes (Author of Life, the Truth, and Being Free)." *Steve Maraboli Quotes (Author of Life, the Truth, and Being Free)*. Better Today Publishing, n.d. Web. 12 Jan. 2017. <https://www.goodreads.com/author/quotes/4491185.Steve_Maraboli>.

Meyer, Joyce. *Battlefield of the Mind: Winning the Battle in Your Mind*. New York, NY: Warner, 2002. Print.

Shaw, George Bernard. "George Bernard Shaw Quotes." *BrainyQuote*. Xplore, n.d. Web. 12 Jan. 2017. <https://www.brainyquote.com/quotes/authors/g/george_bernard_shaw.html>.